I0422092

THE MISADVENTURES

OF ME AND MY UTERUS

MY EXPERIENCES AS
A PERI-MENOPAUSAL WOMAN DEALING
WITH A MEAN SPIRITED UTERUS

BY LAURIE W-J-N

7. Hormones gone wild aka sudden urges to cry and eat chocolate

8. Ablation – ♪ it's electric! ♫

9. Fight like a girl……-If I study hard can I get a better grade?

10. No Womb at the Inn – a hysterectomy

11. Okay – now what?

Introduction:

I just recently realized that in a few short months, I will officially be joining the grey brigade. It is so strange to think about actually being a half century old; it is even stranger to realize that those 50 years have passed faster than a Twinkie at weight watchers. I know that lots of folks fear getting older, – and to be fair, there are lots of struggles and challenges that come with age, but I really do feel like I am having the best time of my life right now. My two beautiful daughters are grown and I have found an incredible partner to spend my life with, so things are really good.

But… some of you knew that but was coming, didn't you? Coming close to 50 also means entering that most dreaded time of a woman's life – Menopause. If you are too young to think about the big M, you can stop reading right now; this book won't mean much to you. If you are the husband or significant other of a woman going through life's greatest change –this book will explain why the woman you love occasionally turns into a raving lunatic. If you are a woman in her late 40's or older, I offer a taste of what to expect, and a reminder that you are not alone.

I share my story, because when I was going through all of this, I wish I'd had someone I could talk to who'd gone through it before me. There were times I felt so alone and scared, and I really needed reassurance from someone who could tell me what to expect. Pregnant women clutch their copies of 'What to Expect When You're Expecting" so think of this as your very own "*What to Expect When Your Uterus Decides to Become Mean and Downright Evil*". This book is not meant to replace medical advice, it's simply me, telling my story in the hopes that it makes you laugh or even better, that it helps you get through any kind of similar health issue.

Chapter 1.

Parts is Parts – a basic female anatomy review

Let's begin with the basics. Inside a woman's body is a very special place that is often called a womb. This miraculous organ is designed to nurture a baby until it is ready to enter the world. People often describe the womb in such a loving way. The medical term for a womb is uterus, but I have rarely heard people describe a uterus in an equally loving way. We woman have a complicated relationship with our uterus. Each month a woman's uterus creates a thick, soft lining full of nutrients for a baby, but then at some point during the month the body realizes that it has been betrayed and that a baby isn't growing, so the uterus decides to punish the woman by violently ripping out this lining and exploding the whole thing out of the body.

Doctors may have a different explanation, but if you have ever suffered from cramps you know that my description is much more accurate. Why is the uterus so angry at women? The answer is simple, God really must be a man, and he is still angry and upset about his first girlfriend breaking up with him, so he is using the uterus to get back at us all. No wait, that's not right, the reason we need a uterus is for the sole purpose of bringing children into this world. When used for its intended the purpose the uterus is a truly remarkable organ that houses, protects and nourishes our offspring. It grows to almost 15 times its normal size just before delivery. It is incredibly strong, it not only protects a baby but it aids in the process of labor, contracting muscles to help push the baby out when ready. Strong, resilient and nurturing, it's also capable of inflicting extreme pain – in other words a uterus is uniquely feminine.

I can still vividly recall every moment of my first daughter's birth. I think most of us who have gone through labor can give a pretty accurate moment by moment account – regardless of whether it was six days ago, six weeks ago, six years ago or even six decades ago. There is something about the act of bringing a child into this world that is embedded into the very fiber of your being. Each one of us has a slightly different story, but there are connecting themes throughout each of our unique versions of childbirth.

My version goes something like this, after wandering the house for at least four hours; growing more anxious with each passing minute, my husband and I decided to jump into the car. Of course, we made it to the hospital much too early (as most people do with their first pregnancy). I then wandered the halls in my highly flattering hospital gown for several hours until the pains were too fast and furious to keep walking. Clutching my stomach as best I could I made it back to my bed and was promptly connected up to more machines than I could count. These machines were all monitoring the health status of the baby. The delivering mom, on the other hand, is clearly monitored by the volume of her screaming, and only when it reaches just the right pitch and intensity do the doctors know that the time to deliver is getting close. My husband at the time was very enthralled by all of these wonderful machines, especially the one that monitored the intensity of my contractions. I can still hear my husband saying "wow that was a big one", as he watched on the monitor – I didn't need a monitor to tell me what I was feeling, it hurt.

Finally after waiting, hooked up to machines, and in pain for what seemed like forever (it was actually only 3 hours or so), the doctor came in to check my progress and instantly everything went into hyper-drive. Nurses were running in and out of the room, setting up equipment, and just as I was struggling to breathe through another big contraction, a nurse asked if I wanted her to set up a mirror so I could watch what was going on. A mirror? To this day I can hear my resounding response, "Ewwww." I didn't want to watch that! I had seen enough during my childbirth classes; the films of live childbirth were almost more than I could take, and I certainly didn't need or want a mirror. I could feel every part of the delivery and I did not need to watch. I'm not sure how I developed my inhibition about my own body, but watching a child come slipping out of my uterus was more than I ever wanted to see.

I don't know if other moms felt the same way. Did other people actually want to look at their babies slipping and sliding and tearing their way out down there? I wanted to retain some privacy and dignity; despite the fact that so much of my childbirth process felt like it was a public event. Nurses continued walking in and out of the room, my doctor, a woman who had seen my 'private parts' on many occasions, was sitting on a small stool at the foot of my bed, giving me directions and doing the things a doctor does during deliveries. Even more nurses were walking in and out, some brought equipment, and some were watching monitors; once the baby arrived, several more staff were taking care of the baby while the doctor finished with me. To this day I cannot tell how many people came and left that hospital room. Privacy and childbirth are mutually exclusive.

So how does this miracle of labor occur? Let's back up and review the basics.

Nothing can induce a round of nervous giggling more than discussions of puberty. Does anyone else remember the awful 'films' that were meant to teach us everything we needed to know about our bodies in grade school? After watching them, I had some basic awareness of the shape of my uterus with its extended fallopian tubes, but the main point I took away from those early films was an overly happy girl horseback riding, even though it was her time of the month. I still can't understand why everyone was so happy about their 'time of the month' but they sure did seem to be smiling a lot.

Having two older sisters and a mother who was fairly open-minded, I grew up with a pretty good knowledge of the basic facts, but I was intrigued by the idea of my own body. Not unlike most girls in Junior High, the author Judy Blume was a vital link in my education of the female body and its systems. "Are you there God, it's me Margaret?" helped me to discover this whole elusive 'period' thing. I related so well the Margaret's angst waiting for her period to finally arrive. I knew that having my period was the way I would be recognized as a woman. Of course later in life we all long for that greatly anticipated period to finally be done with, once and for all. Good riddance to *Aunt Flo*, the *curse* and every other euphemism for my time of the month.

The science of reproduction is pretty simple. As I had taught my students in sixth grade science, all living things reproduce (and yes their response was a series of sounds that resembled "ewww and gross"). The female body is essentially built to make and care for babies. Obviously there is a ton of variation in all of those millions of female bodies on our planet, but we mammals all have pretty much the same basic parts.

Now in case you didn't pay attention to the birds and bees talk that was offered at your school, or if you we were one of the kids who didn't go to the lessons and just sat in the library because your mom didn't want you to hear about all this, let's do a quick review of female anatomy.

Starting with the things that few, if any, men actually know. For women, the reproductive system is located entirely in the pelvis (the area between your hips). The outside or external part of the female reproductive organs is called the **vulva**, which sounds like a foreign car, but is actually the part that covers the opening to the **vagina** and the other reproductive organs which are located inside the body. Skin flaps called the **labia** surround the vaginal opening, not to be confused with Libya, which is a foreign country in the Middle East. Confusion between these two could lead to some interesting challenges. The much acclaimed **clitoris** is located near the front of the vulva, although most men cannot find it – because let's face it, men will not stop and ask for directions.

The internal reproductive organs include the vagina, uterus, fallopian tubes, and ovaries. This is typically where our problems start. Understanding what each of these powerful organs do and where they are located, as well as how they are supposed to work can help when dealing with any issues later.

Your parents probably never used any of these terms, and if you are like me you had sweet little nicknames for most of these when speaking to your own children. At our house we used the term "your privates" to cover all areas 'down there'. Raising two daughters, this terminology seemed like a good way to avoid discussing any intimate topics while reinforcing the idea that NO ONE should be messing around with something that was clearly labeled PRIVATE. You may have learned or used other names for your private parts, but for this section we will just stick with the basic scientific terms.

The vagina has more nicknames than any other part of your female anatomy. It's a muscular, hollow tube that extends from the vaginal opening to the uterus and since it has muscular walls it can expand and contract. This ability to become wider or narrower allows the vagina to accommodate something as slim as a tampon and as wide as a baby. While some women worry that their vaginas might stretch out over time, particularly after popping out a baby or two, it is a muscle, and just like other muscles, with some exercise this muscle can get right back in shape (at least in theory). The vagina's muscular walls are lined with mucous membranes, which keep it protected and moist, and can be incredibly annoying at times, causing the need to always be prepared with panti-liners. As you may already know, the vagina has three main jobs: first and foremost the vagina is necessary and important for sexual intercourse, and naturally, following said intercourse, a vagina is the pathway that a baby takes out of a woman's body during childbirth, and finally, as women are all too aware, the vagina is the route for menstrual blood to flow from the uterus and leave the body.

The vagina connects with the **uterus**, or as it was referred to back-in-the-day, the womb. The place where the vagina and uterus meet is the cervix. The cervix is like a small cap at the top of the vagina. The opening of the cervix is normally very small, but during childbirth, the cervix can expand to allow a baby to pass through. When women are in labor you will often hear numbers relating to the cervix. Doctors use a one through ten numbering system to tell how far open the cervix is and thus how close a women is to pushing out her baby. Having gone through labor, I think a one through ten scream intensity scale might be more accurate, but doctors insist on using the cervix as a guide. Once the cervix is all the way open, or dilated to 10, the baby is ready to come on out, leading to even more screaming.

Next we will review my nemesis, the uterus. Many people have described the shape of the uterus like an upside-down pear, which makes it sound gentle, but as I have learned – there is nothing gentle about it. Like the vagina, it has strong muscular walls; in fact the uterus contains some of the strongest muscles in the female body. These muscles are able to expand and contract to accommodate a growing fetus and then help push the baby out during labor, and by help I mean violently contract and forcible shove the baby out with powerful waves of contractions. The uterus has a thick lining that nourishes and protects the fetus (and trust me you will learn more about this lining later in my story).

At the top of the uterus, two **fallopian** tubes, that look like alien arms connect the uterus to the **ovaries**. The ovaries are two oval-shaped organs that produce, store, and release eggs into the fallopian tubes in the process called **ovulation,** also known as the beginning of monthly torture of women everywhere. It is hard to believe but the fallopian tubes are about as wide as a piece of spaghetti. Within each tube is a tiny passageway no wider than a sewing needle. At the other end of each fallopian tube is a fringed area that wraps around the ovary but doesn't completely attach to it. When an egg pops out of an ovary, tiny little fingers reach out and grab it, much like your children instantly grabbing Eggos out of the toaster, and then the egg enters the fallopian tube. Once in the fallopian tube, tiny hairs in the tube's lining help push the egg down the narrow passageway toward the uterus. Every once in a while the eggs can actually get stuck in the tube, and if by chance a friendly little sperm, with just the right timing, makes his way up the tube, something called an ectopic pregnancy can result.

The ovaries are also part of the endocrine system because they produce female sex hormones such as **estrogen** and **progesterone** and you'll hear lots more about these dastardly hormones later.

As amazing as this sounds – all women have these same parts, even infants have them. When a baby girl is born, her ovaries already contain thousands of eggs, which simply remain there, inactive until the joy of puberty begins. At puberty, the pituitary gland, located in the central part of the brain, starts making hormones that stimulate the ovaries to produce female sex hormones, including estrogen, creating lifelong chaos and turmoil. These hormones cause a girl to begin developing sexually, which also means the start of her monthly release of eggs, and the ever popular menstrual cycle.

Okay, now that many of you are thoroughly embarrassed, the basic biology portion of our book is now completed.

Chapter 2.

Menopause –puberty in reverse

For most women, the stage of your life called menopause happens slowly over several years. I realize this sounds like extended torture, but the good news is not all menopausal symptoms happen all at once. Much like when your body went into puberty, without warning you will begin to experience some interesting or uncomfortable new bodily occurrences. For example, instead of waking up with hair on your underarms, now you get to wake up with weird hairs growing on your chin. Being prepared for puberty is a little different than being prepared for menopause, instead of asking your girl friends to borrow a tampon or sanitary pad because you forgot yours, now you ask your girlfriends if you can stick your head in their freezer.

Perhaps the most well known menopause symptoms for women are hot flashes. These little adventures can happen at any time of the day or night, and they prefer to happen at the most inopportune times. I have a friend who refers to these little blessed events as her own personal trip to the tropics, which is actually a quite fitting description for the sudden feeling that you are drowning inside a hot humid swamp of some kind. While doctors do know these exciting adventures in sweat have something to do with declining levels of hormones, they are not completely sure exactly how and why these hot flashes occur.

For me, these free sauna passes actually start in one specific spot, my face or neck, only to slowly migrate across my entire body. The really good news is the once I am completely drenched in sweat, after 4 or 5 minutes it actually starts to go away. Until I get another one at the next most inopportune time.

Another prominent feature of menopause are frequent headaches, this also has something to do with the changing levels of hormones in your body. Even women who are not prone to regular headaches seem to have more of them during this fantastic adventure of menopause. My headaches got so severe that I went to the doctor and she ordered a MRI scan on my brain just to make sure I didn't have a tumor. While I was pleased with my doctor for being so thorough, I can't say it made me feel any better to know that with no significant results from the MRI, the likely cause of headaches was just menopause, the gift that keeps on giving.

One of the most dreaded symptoms of menopause for women is weight gain. As your body enters menopause, your metabolism slows down and the weight can begin to add up, particularly in the middle section of your body, giving your shape that lovely barrel effect that so many women desire. Some try valiantly to ward off the weight gain by frantic attempts at diet and exercise, but often this is not entirely successful. This weight gain is also a contributing factor to other health issues. Women in menopause are struggling against their own body, to lose weight.

The most notorious symptom of menopause might be the mood swings and irritability – but since we have already mentioned hair growth in unwanted places, hot flashes, headaches and weight gain – is it really any surprise that women going through menopause are irritable? Now most women have had their own experiences with occasional moodiness or irritability, some women struggle with severe PMS or pre-menstrual syndrome. I am very sorry to tell these women that these symptoms do not go away with menopause, they actually get slightly worse, until your hormone levels decrease enough, or you get senile enough, to not care anymore.

Doctors generally agree that a woman is officially in menopause once her monthly periods have stopped for a year or longer, which is the only menopause symptom that I was actually looking forward to.

Going through the period of time called peri-menopause means that you are lucky enough to suffer through some or all of the typical symptoms of menopause and still be menstruating on a regular basis. Yes, my friends, you are still technically fertile and functioning, even as your reproductive system starts to slowly shut down. This constant struggle between two worlds is the crux of the dilemma, your body is literally fighting a civil war, and you, my friend, are on the list of casualties.

Chapter 3

Spring-loaded Uterus (and other forms of birth control)

Without attempting to go into an exposé of my past sexual exploits (believe me – they're not that exciting), I can say I have tried most forms of birth control. I was born in the turbulent sixties and grew up in the seventies with older siblings and a Mom who was more progressive than most, so I can safely say I was part of the new female liberation generation. That did not give me freedom or license to sleep around by any means, but it meant that it was my job to deal with birth control as an independent woman. Remember – I was still a child in the seventies, so while free love and all that stuff may have existed in San Francisco, it was not alive and well in the suburbs of Tucson, Arizona. We didn't have 'friends with benefits'. A girl who slept around was still considered a slut (although a guy who slept around was considered a stud – an unfair situation that still lingers to this day).

When I was younger, like many girls I went on 'the pill' and used that effectively until I was ready to start a family. I think I started on the pill somewhere between sixteen or seventeen years old. Yes, my mom did know about me going on the pill, well eventually. She wasn't really happy about me being on the pill, but she would have been even less happy to have me come home pregnant.

I might be giving too much away about my age (and let's face it, the fact that I discuss menopause in the book clearly throws me under the bus right there), but I don't remember any of us worrying about STD's and AIDS the way kids do now. It was always assumed the girl would 'handle everything.' I especially liked the pill packages with the placebo pills. I was never the kind of person who could skip a week and then get right back on track. I needed that daily routine. Too bad we didn't have smart phones back then so I could have just set a daily reminder – it would have eliminated many of my stressful moments when I realized I had forgotten to take my pill. I sat there, like most co-eds, struggling with the question of whether I could or would get pregnant, and if I doubled up, would that make it better? For the most part, the pill seemed to work fairly well for me through high school and college.

I was not very promiscuous (I told you I wasn't that exciting), sleeping around was something that loose girls did, and I was not one of 'those' girls. I had a few serious boyfriends and eventually things got … ummm, even more serious, but in general I would say I had pretty limited experience compared with many of my college friends. I met my husband when I was 20 and got married at the ridiculously tender age of 21. Before you start to lecture me on all the reasons why that was such a horrible idea, it's too late to do anything about that now and I did stay married for 23 years until his death. When we were first married I stayed on the pill so we could finish school, get jobs and get settled in a home of our own before we even thought about having any children.

At the age of 24, my husband and I decided it was time for me to go off the pill. People asked if we were trying to have a baby and our adorable and entirely unhelpful response was that we were "not trying not to" but given that I had obviously inherited my mother's overly fertile genes, I became pregnant almost overnight. I later learned from someone that after having been on the pill for an extended period of time, you are highly likely to get pregnant right away. Well it worked. Ready or not we were about to have a baby. I had a beautiful healthy baby girl and enjoyed being a mom.

As far as birth control goes, the pill had served its purpose well in my early years. I was young and healthy and monogamous, so the pill was a great alternative for me at the time. Deciding what to do for birth control after the baby was a harder choice than I realized. I did not really want to go back on the pill. I knew there could be many possible complications with long term use of the pill.

After the pregnancy I decided to use my mother's old tried and true form of birth control – the diaphragm. My mother's stories of birth control are legendary, including one about how she never knew that a diaphragm should be re-fitted after each pregnancy, which according to my mother resulted in more than one additional pregnancy. In addition to her insights about the use of a diaphragm, I learned from my mother that the rhythm method is very effective at achieving pregnancy.

For those of you not familiar with it, a diaphragm is a small round silicone dome shaped cup that goes into your vagina and fits over the cervix, it is literally a barrier which is intended to keep those pesky little sperm from entering the uterus and meeting up with an egg. The diaphragm is considered more effective if it is used with a chemical spermicide (a gel which is designed to kill any sperm it comes in contact with). Not only is it slightly awkward to insert the diaphragm, but it is also extremely awkward to remove the diaphragm after you are done. The good news is that you are not only allowed to, but you are expected to wait awhile before removal, to help the spermicide do its job of mass homicide to the sperm in your vagina.   Some people have problems with sensitivity to the spermicide, but fortunately, that never seemed to be an issue for me.

After a slight learning curve (yes pun intended – it was tough getting that slippery disk into place at first) I was successfully using the diaphragm until my husband and I began discussing the idea of adding to our family, and we were not in agreement. This dispute went back and forth for a number of weeks, I made it clear that for me having a family was children and not a single child. There were tears and arguments. He seemed pretty adamant about not having more kids and I was every bit as adamant about having another. This, my friends, is where my story takes a slight turn and shows my deceptive nature. I was unwavering about wanting another child, being a mom was deeply embedded in my DNA.

I want to preface this next section by saying I do have my daughter's permission to share this part of my story. She laughed out loud when I admitted this story to her and I think she takes a certain amount of pride in knowing how much I wanted her and what lengths I was willing to go to in order to have her. At least, I hope so!

This argument between my husband and I went on for several weeks. I was continuing to use my diaphragm and one day I had a brilliant moment of clarity (at least from my point of view) and I realized that diaphragms have been known to fail (refer back to my mother's stories). I recalled having seen some other deceptive women in various Hollywood movies who wanted to get pregnant, so I took it upon myself to 'help this argument along' and I took out my diaphragm and proceeded to put several small holes in it with a pin. These holes were not visible, but I had faith that those brave little swimmers would find them. Not to belabor the point (again, pun intended) but we wound up having another beautiful daughter. I never did admit my deception to my husband, but I can assure you he loved both of his daughters and was happy they had both entered the world. It was a decision that I will never regret.

After the birth of my second child I decided to try something new called a Norplant. It was a quick simple procedure in a doctor's office. I watched with awe and slight revulsion while they shoved these tiny little tubes just under the skin of my upper arm, designed to slowly release hormones that would prevent pregnancy, pretty much like a longer term internal version of the pill. I kept the Norplant tubes in for over a year, but the odd feeling of those plastic tubes under my skin was just too strange, and I kept wondering about the strange hormones inside those tubes, so I had them removed.

This left me without any birth control, and I did want another baby someday, but not right away. I had to find something, non-permanent, that would work for me. I tried a few temporary methods, including a weird sponge device that you could buy at any drug store. The idea was the sponge would both absorb and help block sperm like a diaphragm and it had spermicide in it to kill as many sperm cells as possible. It was easy enough, but I wasn't confident it was really the best choice; I knew I needed something easier and long lasting. I am not the kind of person who likes to remember something each day, I want to simply get it and promptly forget about it. I also don't like to have to prepare to be intimate. This led me to an IUD. I had heard so many urban legend horror stories about terrible cramps and periods, but I went ahead and gave it a try and it worked so well that I kept mine in for over 10 years without any problems.

An IUD, or inter uterine device, is inserted into your uterus by a doctor. While not too pleasant an experience, I did not have any problems with the procedure. It went quickly and for me, and after some initial cramps getting used to the device, I had very little change to my monthly cycle and period pains. For the most part, my cramps have always been manageable – they are annoying, but not debilitating like someone suffering from endometriosis (a condition where the lining of the uterus, also known as the endometrium, is inflamed and this causes more severe and painful monthly cycles).

My gynecological life remained fairly unremarkable for the next 10 years, but then everything changed in an instant; my husband died and everything else in my life changed too. Honestly, I really am not quite sure why I felt the need to remove the device after my husband died (his death was sudden and unexpected – a story for another book). I think I was over-thinking everything at that point, being a relatively young widow, I was feeling overwhelmed and trying to control everything that I could, because my life felt so out of control. My IUD was still there and it wasn't bothering anyone, but as I said I was overthinking this. I had read something about the lifespan of an IUD device being only 7-10 years, and I knew I had mine for over 10 years, so being the rule follower that I am, I went to the doctor and had the IUD removed.

And then I started dating…

Being single again after so many years, and being in my mid-forties, I was completely unprepared to think about sex, let alone contraception, but I knew that I needed some form of birth control if I was going to enter the dating world. Since I was in my forties, I was fairly confident in choosing something permanent. It was sad to realize that I would never have more babies, but to be honest at a certain point in your life, it is a relief to realize that the only babies in your future will be grandchildren. I know it is a tough decision for many, but for me it seemed like the right time.

I went to the doctor and asked for advice. We talked about various options and when my doctor suggested the Essure, I thought it sounded like a great idea. I was already a big fan of IUD's, but many of the new ones now came with hormones, and I wasn't crazy about adding extra hormones to my body.

The Essure was a simple device that was permanent and could be done in an office visit. Simple. No hormones. No more babies. No major surgery. Covered by insurance......I was sold, so I made my appointment. It really was as simple as they said. I felt a weird slight pinching feeling as they passed each spring through my cervix and up into each of the fallopian tubes. They did say to expect some cramping, but to be honest I have had periods that were worse than the cramps from the Essure. The doctor did want me to follow up with a procedure to ensure the coils had created the necessary scar tissue to prevent the eggs from passing through the fallopian tubes, by getting a procedure, but the only place that would do the follow up was over 40 miles away and I simply didn't bother to go (I know – pretty strange for a rule follower like me, but I think I was going through a rebellious period). I was banking on the fact that I was in my mid-forties, and I was pretty confident that my eggs were done or at least fading fast. I think I was underestimating my body's attempts at fertility. Clearly my uterus was not done trying to nourish eggs, which led to the struggles I suffered.

I have always been open and honest with my daughters, so when I told my younger daughter what I had done and explained about the procedure, she giggled and exclaimed that I now had a spring-loaded uterus. We both still describe my uterus that way to this day. Having an Essure as my birth control is simple, the majority of the time I don't even know it is there, but I did notice a new sensation – I could actually feel when I was ovulating. Yes, I know it sounds weird, but once an eggs was released, I could feel slight sharp cramps as the egg tried to get through the tubes and were stopped by the springs and scar tissue. At least that's what I could feel based on where I got these little occasional sharp cramps just a few days before my cycle.

I am a firm believer in listening to your body. I think we are much more attuned to our unique systems than any doctor could be and we need to pay attention to what our body is telling us. These were very specific cramps, sharp and not lasting more than 1 or 2 days at the most. They always happened just a week or so before my periods. At this point birth control seems like a moot point, but it was a big deal for me at the time. The Essure might not be right for everyone, and certainly it is not an option for anyone who might still want to get pregnant, but it worked well for me.

I did manage to survive mid-life dating (and that really is a story for another book) and I met a wonderful man named Peter who is happy and fun and full of life, and he has been such a supportive partner through all of my many misadventures.

Chapter 4

What's normal anyway? Spot is a dog not a lifestyle

Getting older means many things, like being invited to AARP, and it means all of that messy menopause stuff, which no one wants to talk about it, and believe me it's not pretty. The good news is a woman's menstrual cycle tends to shorten and get more regular with age. The bad news; menopause messes everything up – including your monthly cycle. I had heard about and experienced an occasional hot flash and some of the other odd side effects of menopause, but I was under the impression that one day your period would just go away (and wouldn't that be wonderful). If that sounds too good to be true – it is. Your menstrual cycle doesn't just go out with a whimper – it fights tooth and nail to hang on until the last possible moments – making your life miserable for as long as possible, or at least that's what happened for me.

Being a generally organized individual, I tried to keep a record of my monthly cycle. I figured this would help me know when to expect my monthly friend – thus helping me plan when to go away for romantic weekends, etc. As I was diligently recording, I noticed a disturbing pattern. My menstrual cycle was going wacky, shortening to almost 10 days apart – which as you can imagine was seriously annoying, so I went to the Doctor and asked if this was normal (an obviously silly question for anyone who has gone through menopause, because absolutely nothing is normal about it). Her response was, "It's probably nothing; it's probably just your hormones fluctuating as you get nearer to menopause". Ugh, she was right, I was getting close to menopause, closer to being old and gray (but at least I can keep buying my Clairol root touch up kit). Was this what I had to look forward to? I thought those pesky periods would go away, not come more often. She did suggest that we do an ultra sound "just to be sure', although at the time, I didn't know what we were trying to be sure about.

With school almost ending and plenty going on in my life, the ultrasound got put onto the back burner, on the pile of things "I was planning to get to". I was still tracking my crazy erratic cycle and doing my best to get through another school year. On the very last day of school my period started, and then it never stopped. I felt like this was a bad omen for my summer. Every single day I was spotting and when I finally looked closely at the calendar, I realized that I had endured 20 straight days of fairly heavy spotting. At this point I was tremendously frustrated, so I found my ultra sound referral and made my appointment as soon as possible. Then I waited for the appointment, and kept spotting. I don't know how other women feel about this, but I find even one or two days of spotting to be bothersome, so spotting for more than 20 days straight was seriously annoying, to put it mildly. It was summertime in Phoenix. Yes, picture hot weather, cute shorts and me – wearing pads every single day, because spotting is not enough to need a tampon, and without something I would be in trouble. At this point I was feeling cranky, wondering if I could go swimming, and wondering if this would ever end.

According to the U.S. Office of Women's Health, an average woman's monthly cycle is 28 days, but menstrual cycles can range anywhere from 21 to 35 days. The rise and fall of hormones controls the monthly cycle; hormone levels rise to help prepare the uterine lining for pregnancy. As we all know from the countless tampon and panti-liner commercials, periods can be light, moderate, heavy, or in my case later that summer, Category 4 Storm Surge levels. The length of an average period also varies. Most periods last from 3 to 5 days longs, but anywhere from 2 to 7 days is normal – so it is safe to assume that 40 days straight of bleeding not only puts me in a category that rivals Noah and the flood, but it was NOT considered normal.

I want to take a minute here to discuss something serious. ALL doctors will tell you that any excessive or prolonged bleeding can be serious, particularly for women who have already gone through menopause. It is extremely important to go and get any abnormal bleeding checked out.

Chapter 5

Nothing says fun like a

transvaginal ultrasound

As most women already know, having to deal with 'female' problems usually means sacrificing your privacy. Upon arriving at the ultrasound appointment, I didn't really have any idea what to expect. I was drinking as much water as I could possible swallow without getting sick, because the directions were very clear to drink water and NOT use the restroom for one hour prior to the procedure. The girl on the phone made a point of telling me three times that my bladder needed to be full.   Well at this point my eyelids were floating; I had to pee so badly it hurt. I was horribly uncomfortable and of course it felt like forever before they called me back. I followed a technician through a maze of tunnel like hallways to a small dressing room and she told me to get undressed, "Everything from the waist down". These were directions I got very familiar with during the remainder of the summer at all of my subsequent appointments and procedures.

I got undressed and put on the ill-fitting and very embarrassing gown, walked partway back down the maze of tunnel like hallways, (did I mention I was wearing the ill-fitting and embarrassing gown?), and I got on the table as directed. At this point, the information fliers in the waiting room explained that "You will feel slight pressure while a sonographer moves a hand-held device". Now let me remind you, my bladder was incredibly full - so it is more than slight pressure, I was so worried about peeing on this lady's table that I did't even have time to worry about what results she might be finding. She was pushing this cold tool across my belly and yes she was pushing in hard in certain spots. Finally, mercifully, she told me to go to the restroom before we finished the rest of the procedure. I had to pee so badly I didn't even ask what the rest of the procedure was.

For those of you who have not had the privilege of a transvaginal ultrasound (yes, that's the one in the news that a bunch of male politicians want to require women to require women to undergo, which instantaneously makes me want to shove something up their private parts and see if they like it), they are a unique experience. After perhaps the most wonderful use of a restroom that I have ever had, I walked back in the room and got back up on the table and the technician pulled out a HUGE plastic object that looked disturbingly like a vibrator on steroids that was carefully covered in plastic adding nothing positive to its menacing appearance. She explained that she would be looking "internally" at my uterus now. It is hard to imagine how awkward this whole situation was, unless you have experienced it (which explains why I want to offer some first had experience to these male politicians who think nothing of making ridiculous laws that require these of women).

The technician was trying to be very pleasant, but let's face it – there is NOTHING pleasant about this experience. I was sitting very still and trying my very best to ignore what was going on below my waist, when I looked over at the technician and realized that she seemed to be slightly scowling. This was NOT a good sign; she repositioned the instrument numerous times and seemed to be concentrating heavily on the screen. Now I could have assume she was just diligent in her work, but since she had been attempting awkward social chattiness earlier, I was certain this was not a good thing. I was now more concerned with what she was seeing than the horrendously ungainly position that I was in.

As she repositioned the vibrator-probe instrument, she tapped and clicked her computer repeatedly and scowled some more, I was not feeling very positive. Finally she told me, we were finished and I should go get dressed. She very politely explained that my doctor would have the results and would give me a call. I was distracted as I get dressed, knowing that I now had to patiently wait for the doctor to call, and I am NOT a patient person.

After a few days of restless waiting, I began to do some research, it's what I always do when I face something new and potentially scary. Knowledge is power. My first line of defense has always been to research and learn more about what I am facing. Sometimes that knowledge can be scary to face, but in the long run it always helps to know what you are dealing with. I sat and did google search queries about heavy spotting, frequent periods, etc. The research turned up mixed results, so I didn't feel any more informed. I did however feel like something was not right.

That gut feeling, women's intuition, whatever 'it' is, I have it, I always have – however sometimes I choose to ignore it. Well that feeling that said there is something going on, it was right, I received a call from the doctor's office saying, "we need you to come in" (at this exact moment I can hear the orchestra background in my head playing scary music). If you have ever had a doctor call and say we need you to come in, you know how intimidating this sentence can be.

The doctor's assistant proceeded to explain that I had something called "a thickening of the uterine lining" and I need something called an endometrial biopsy. According to the doctor's assistant, this is a pretty simple procedure where the doctor will scrape a few cells from the lining of my uterus, so we can get them checked out. I scheduled my appointment, but it was over a week away. Just to re-state, I have never been a very patient person, so to simply sit and wait for this procedure, and see what kind of cells they find is not exactly something anyone would be good at, and I am more impatient than most. I was driving myself crazy, reading online about a thickened uterine lining, and wondering what this might mean. Getting more and more apprehensive about the biopsy procedure with each passing day. Having several days to wait for this procedure was probably the worst thing for me. More google searches. More results. Now for the scary part, if they find atypical cells during the biopsy, it could be endometrial cancer. Yup, I said the C word. Even worse than the M word, much worse.

There is just something about the word cancer that reduces grown men and women into scared little toddlers. It's a cloud of dread that hangs over anyone who says the word, let alone actually struggles with the disease. I am not typically a fearful person, most people would describe me as optimistic, so when faced with the big C, I really struggled with it. I felt like there was no one I could talk to, except my amazing fiancé, but even then I knew that sharing what I had learned would be difficult. Knowing Peter, I knew he had already done his research too. As we talked about it, he tried to be reassuring, but I could see the fear in his eyes. I can't imagine how he felt, having lost many family members to cancer, it was not something he remotely wanted to think about.

I knew that if there was a problem, I could not have been taken care of better by anyone. He was so kind and caring and surprisingly patient with me. So the waiting for the next week or two was the hardest part, because once I knew if there was an issue I could deal with my fear and face it head on - because that's what I do. If it was bad news, there were still lots of reason to be optimistic, even though endometrial cancer is the most common gynecologic malignancy in the United States, and the fourth most common female malignancy, the **Overall survival is excellent** since 75% of patients have the disease confined to the uterus. See what I mean, I am usually very optimistic, but unless I know what I am facing – it's hard to deal with it.

Despite still waiting to get the test, I was enjoying drifting along this summer in a casual, no rush, no worries manner, or at least trying to. Laying out by the pool, working a little, trying to get inspired to work or to write, mostly reading books, watching movies and just wasting time. I was doing my best to just relax, but this whole *endometrial hyperplasia* was really throwing me off balance and I was focusing on it way more than I should. When I found myself getting overly anxious, I would remind myself that that even the worst case scenario means removing my uterus and then it's taken care of. I just needed to change my focus onto the cool fun summer plans I had - and just let go of needing to control things - yeah right!

Chapter 6.

Endometrial hyperplasia and other aliens

Endometrial Hyperplasia is simply a fancy medical term for a thickening of the uterine lining. Basically my uterus keeps getting ready for a monthly period, but for some reason is not doing a good job of shedding the lining each month, causing it to build up. Most doctors believe the buildup is due to an increased level of hormones.   It's this buildup that has the doctors worried, because apparently when uterine lining cells are just sitting around, much like teenagers, they have a tendency to get into trouble. This is why the doctor wants to take a closer look at the cells, but since they are way up in the uterus, they are a little but harder to get to.

For those of you who have never experienced one, let me assure you, an endometrial biopsy is not fun. Once again I was undressed from the waist down in an ugly and embarrassing gown, and I was sitting on an exam table with my most private parts exposed to the doctor and her assistant. At least the doctor and her assistant were both women, this was not the case for many of the other exams and procedures I later went through. The doctor was awesome though, very open and honest, she took her time explaining my other test results and she told me exactly what to expect with the procedure. Apparently my uterine lining was over 21mm, which is extremely thick – a normal uterine lining is half that much, and someone in menopause should be even thinner than that, so it was obviously a problem. She also explained what the possible results of the biopsy might be, and the likely treatments that would accompany each one. This information wasn't totally a surprise since I had spent some time researching.

If it was found cancerous the likely result would be a hysterectomy. I wasn't extremely bothered by the idea of a hysterectomy, I obviously had no plans to have any more children (remember my spring loaded uterus), but let's face it, there is never a good time to do surgery. The more I began to think about the possibilities, the more I was freaking myself out. On the bright side, more than likely, even with a confirmation of cancerous cells, I would only need a hysterectomy and no chemo or radiation. Even the words chemotherapy and radiation are terrifying. It was easy to be overwhelmed by any or all of this.

Back to the procedure at hand, using her special tool for female parts, the speculum (ladies you are familiar with this one from your yearly pap smear), the doctor began the procedure. She used an awful clamp like thing to hold on to and open my cervix up enough for her to get a sample of the uterine lining. It was not the worst pain I have even felt, but it was a nasty pinching feeling, followed by a weird sensation of pressure as the doctor scraped the inside of my uterus to gather some cells. Apparently, it is important to get cells from several different areas inside of your uterus, so the procedure lasted longer than I wanted it to. Finally she took off the nasty clamp like tool, and said she was finished. I wish I could say I was relieved, but then she explained it could take up to two full weeks to get the test results. Two full weeks of wondering what was going on inside of my uterus. Did I already mention I am NOT a patient person?

As the doctor and her assistant left the room and I began to get dressed, I was alone with my thoughts swirling around in my head. One moment I was optimistic, saying to myself, "This is nothing". The next moment I was almost paralyzed with fear at even the idea of cancer. I assume this is a common feeling for most people who have to go through something like this.

Before I could even get into the car, Peter was calling to check up on me. He has been amazing. He was so patient, and we sat and talked at length about all of this. We had decided not to tell anyone else until there is some 'actual' news to tell. Having Peter here to reassure me was so great, but I worried about him, he has had such an ugly family history with cancer, his mother and father both died from cancer, I knew this freaked him out a bit too – even if he was acting like he was handling everything just fine.   Now we have nothing left to do but wait. I was pretty much fearing and planning for the worst, but mildly hopeful for the best.

Let's face it - getting older isn't for sissies, but this week has been ridiculous. I have been crampy from the biopsy and not very motivated for the past few days. I think the stress of everything is stealing my energy. The really good news is that I haven't been bleeding heavily, just mild cramps off and on since the biopsy. Fortunately, I have plans to be going on vacation with Peter next week. I think a chance to just get away from all of this will be wonderful.

I had been asking for ages to go kayaking in San Diego, they have a cool guided trip to these sea caves and I was psyched to see them. I know kayaking isn't really Peter's thing, but I just love it, and he was feeling so bad about everything that was going on so he arranged a business trip to San Diego and Los Angeles that I could come along with and we made plans to do the kayaking. I was really looking forward to that. Anytime at the ocean is excellent – I think the ocean has magical healing powers for your soul.

So my week began, tagging along with Peter while he visits his customer sites in California. We had it all planned, a day in San Diego before heading up to his favorite place-Huntington beach. Seemed like a perfect plan except for one thing - MY MEAN UTERUS! The trip started out really nicely, after a small argument about hotels we decided to splurge on a beautiful place in La Jolla with an ocean view. I am pretty sure my nasty mood was the deciding factor in choosing the over-priced hotel with an ocean view. We went out for a lovely romantic dinner with a view of the ocean from our table. We strolled along the waterfront holding hands and taking pictures. Our reservation was all set for kayaking, and I was really enjoying the day with Peter. I had tried my best to put my uterus out of my mind and just enjoy the trip.

The next morning I was spotting a little and slightly crampy, I wondered if I might be starting my period (my cycle has been so nuts lately I had no idea when to expect it) so I prepared as best I could with a tampon & we headed to the kayaks. Peter tried, but decided it really wasn't for him. I had wondered if that might happen- that's why I reserved two singles instead of a tandem kayak. It was so much fun, that I actually got to forget about everything and just enjoy the experience. We kayaked out to some caves and through some cool kelp beds. We saw sea lions. It was a beautiful sunny day. I was feeling so happy, but when we were done and returning to the beach, I had that 'uh-oh' feeling and told Peter I needed a store and a restroom right away. Sure enough, I was big time bleeding. I have never had such a heavy period in my life, not even the bleeding after childbirth compared with this. It didn't slow down at all, cramps and massive un-ending bleeding. I was wearing a pad and a super plus tampon and needing to change every single hour. I knew this wasn't normal. I bought a big box of super plus tampons and I knew I was in big trouble when I asked Peter to find a drug store the next day to buy more. We tried to go out to dinner and I had the use the restroom before we ate, during the meal and after we finished, and I still had to rush to the restroom when we got back to the hotel room. Needless to say this was not the most romantic trip we have ever taken. I decided to call the doctor because all of this bleeding seemed pretty excessive.

Peter went to work and I was sitting alone in a hotel room waiting for the doctor to call back. I would rather have been out on the beach, but having to run to the restroom every hour to change, makes hanging at the beach not as fun as I had hoped. At this point my frustration level was extreme. I wasn't as worried about the idea of cancer; I just wanted my dam uterus to be out so I could stop bleeding and try to be normal. I sat in the hotel room pouting because I was unhappy about all of it. I was upset about the timing and how it was really messing up our fun California vacation - let's face it, a woman who is bleeding heavily is not a very fun partner. Peter was worried about me, so he wasn't having much fun either. At that point, I decided, I don't care how badly I am bleeding, I am going down to the beach!

Chapter 7.

Hormones gone wild aka sudden urges to cry and eat chocolate

It's the dreaded change of life. Not discussed in mixed company – it's that time when women go wildly insane for short periods of time, or at least more insane than usual. Peri-menopause, it may sound exotic, but those going through it know the chaos it can bring, and in general things just get more difficult and complicated. There are hundreds of books written about menopause. Simply put, your body has decided that it's no longer the right time to have a baby so its starts shutting that whole thing down.

Shutting down reproduction starts with your body not making as much of the hormones estrogen and progesterone, which regulate all of your female reproduction and many other things that you may not be aware of. With lower hormone levels, your body slows down and stops menstruation (or at least it's supposed to – but I guess my uterus hadn't gotten the message). These hormones also help regulate your metabolism, which can be a problem for most women.

This whole menopause thing has been a serious challenge to my lifelong weight issues. I have been overweight most of my adult life. Not seriously obese – just overweight like most of America. The hormonal and metabolic changes in menopause cause your body to literally slow down, and this mean less calories are required and those calories that you do eat are not processed as efficiently, causing weight gain particularly around the middle section of the body. This has been absolutely crushing for me. Remember I said I have been overweight most of my adult life, despite having saddlebags and a larger than necessary rear end, I have almost always had a somewhat hourglass figure – albeit somewhat thicker in the bottom half of the glass. With the changes in menopause I now have a tummy pooch. I detest tummy pooches. Not only do I have this pooch, but overall my weight is steadily creeping up. This is not something any woman would be happy about. In addition, my age along with the additional weight has made it harder to go and workout like I did 5 or even 10 years ago.

It is a terrible paradox, knowing that the extra weight puts me at greater risk for endometrial and other cancers, but the extra weight makes it harder to find the necessary motivation to go workout and loose the weight. And on top of all that, the hormones of menopause are literally working against any weight loss efforts on my part. This seems like a cruel and unusual form of punishment.

Once I do muster up the necessary motivation to go and work out I face even more hormonal nightmares. Many of you have heard about hot flashes. Getting a hot flash is not as horrendous as many people suggest, but it is awkward and uncomfortable. The sudden and intense sweatbox that is your body, radiating heat and literally dripping in sweat. Now picture a trip to the gym to walk on the treadmill, lift some weight for the ever important and bone strengthening weight bearing exercises, and maybe hop on the bicycle. Normally these activities would induce some sweat, but add in peri-menopause and fluctuating levels of hormones and now these adventures are sure to induce world class levels of sweat pouring forth from your body. If simply walking upstairs induces a hot flash, jumping on a treadmill is an all-out invitation for your body to go thermonuclear. I find myself looking around to see if anyone notices that I am hotter than the core in *The China Syndrome*.

Working out is not the only area where these evil hormones wreak havoc. I have nightly epic battles with bedding. My evening almost always starts with one of my unwelcome hot flashes. Living in Arizona I am used to the heat, but not the drenching of sweat that comes with each hot flash. I often have to ask, is it hot in here or just me. An Arizona summer is a lot like one of my hot flashes, but for me it is most definitely NOT a dry heat. Almost anything can trigger a hot flash. Did I have a glass of wine? For me red wine is much more likely to trigger a good hot flash. Something sweet to eat – a hot flash. Any physical exertion, like bringing the laundry upstairs, a hot flash. No reason at all, a hot flash. Once it's time for bed I head upstairs, I turn on the air conditioning and the fan and simply lay there for a few minutes as the heat abates. Not surprisingly when I have finally turned off my internal heater, I am drenched and now I'm freezing cold with the a/c and fan blowing on me so I have to snuggle under the covers, which will create a nice warm feeling until the next exciting hot flash when I have to violently throw off the covers because I am boiling and now sweating again. Even the sweating in menopause is different. For some reason now, in addition to everywhere else, the sweating is happening between my breasts. This is an unpleasant place to sweat. This nightly battle rages on for all women lucky enough to have their own adventures in peri-menopause.

Adding the joys of peri-menopause to my uterine struggles and I was pretty much a total mess at this point. It had been a very interesting week. After bleeding profusely for two straight days, I realized I was really bleeding an excessive amount (let's just say I visited more public restrooms than I will ever care to see again and going through a super plus tampon per hour). I decided I had to call the doctor - of course being away in Huntington beach didn't make things any easier, so I was explaining all of this to my doctor's assistant, "um, yes well I have been bleeding so much that I have to get a new superplus tampon each hour." (And yes it is weird to discuss bleeding with a guy over the phone, did he even know the difference between a regular and super tampon?). The doctor called in a prescription, so I filled it, and picked up some recommended high potency iron due to all of my blood loss in the past few days.

I look inside the prescription bag and try to figure out what she wants me to take. The medicine is Norethindrone, which is a progesterone hormone, and from what I read on various internet health sites, it is commonly prescribed for bleeding. I have to say those package inserts full of disclaimers are NOT very comforting - my package basically said don't take this, but if you do, there a bazillion side effects - awesome! No, really, it causes: nausea, vomiting, headache, dizziness, mood swings, trouble sleeping, weight gain/loss (and with my luck lately I'm pretty sure mine will be the gain one), acne, breast swelling/tenderness, change in sexual interest, unwanted hair growth (really- is there usually wanted hair growth?), or hair loss may occur, and those are not even the serious side effects. The package urged me to call my doctor if any of these serious side effects occurred; frequent/burning/painful urination, yellowing eyes/skin, dark patches on the skin or face, serious (possibly fatal) problems from blood clots (e.g., heart attack, stroke, blood clots in the lungs or legs, blindness). Well, I was officially freaked out, so far so good, but I still had no news from the biopsy (translation - already scared & anxious) and now I was scared about the effects of taking hormones (even more scared & anxious).

As I began taking the progesterone, I noticed my hemorrhage level of bleeding starting to slow down after only one day. It's like a miracle drug. I finally didn't have to literally run to the bathroom every hour. My bleeding had slowed way down, until it was more like the lighter days of a normal period – a little more than spotting but nowhere near the chaotic and frustrating pattern of earlier in the week. The not as fun news was that I still had not heard anything from the biopsy, this looming potentially scary news was just hanging in the air, but I guess I can be grateful for the crazy bleeding – at least it gave me something else to focus on.

Distraction is actually a very effective coping technique.

The only major challenge with the hormone was that it was making me really anxious. I don't know if it was a physical reaction to the drug or a psychological reaction to taking this unwanted pill and all the risks that come along with it. I was more tearful, I was restless, and I was having trouble concentrating. In short I was a mess. Peter, unfortunately, took the brunt of all of this emotional turmoil. Every time I would pick up the prescription bottle, I would look at it as if it were public enemy number one. I knew I wanted to stop the insane bleeding, so the pill was necessary, but I was not happy about taking it. I knew I didn't want to stay on this medicine for very long.

The bright side of the pill beginning to work was that I was finally able to go down to the pool - YES I said pool!!!! Because I actually could go down with just a tampon and stay for an hour or two, what a big change from just a few days before. It is amazing how much we can forget to be grateful for the basics in life, when they have been temporarily taken away. Having all this craziness really did help me to appreciate the little things.

Well we started heading home and I was actually happy to get back to my safe and cozy house. It was an interesting trip to say the least. I was surprised, but I really did have fun on the trip – despite the crazy misadventures of a mean-spirited uterus, or maybe even a little bit because of it. Peter and I actually laughed about the hourly struggles to find a restroom and the other chaos and turmoil, and somehow we managed to find a way to go on a romantic walk along the pier and he was so excited to take me to his favorite places in Huntington Beach.

As we drove home Peter and I spent some time talking about everything, I was able to share all of my fears about taking nasty hormones with all of their evil side-effects, but also how grateful I was that the hormones had finally curtailed my out of control bleeding. We both got a chance to share our feels and feel supported by each other. I am so amazed at what a wonderful relationship I have found with him, not many guys would really understand or care about most of this, but he just patiently listened to me and offered advice when he could. Mostly he was so reassuring, he was so firm in his belief that everything would be fine and that we would get through all of this and look back and laugh. To be perfect honest, I had already been laughing a great deal – it was pretty much a laugh or cry situation, and I prefer laughing.

Chapter 8

Ablation – ♪it's electric! ♫

Literally as I was in the car on the way back home, I finally got the phone call from the doctor's office. Rather than make me feel better - it added even more stress and confusion. The doctor's assistant said the results came back normal (*and I can only guess that means no cancer, since having all of these procedures is anything but NORMAL*). Then she went on to explain that if I am still having bleeding issues that I should schedule an ablation or a D&C. Unfortunately she did not elaborate on either procedure, and my head was spinning. What is the difference? Why do I want one of these? What about the hysterectomy? Even if there is no cancer now, is there still a chance of developing it later? I was completely overwhelmed at this point, and talking to a health assistant who isn't really qualified to give me any of these answers, so I made an appointment with the doctor and she hung up. This left me trying to understand all of the options on my own. I knew that I DIDN'T want to continue on hormones for any length of time. I was still bleeding, and cramping, and very scared.

Just the thought that my uterus had cancerous or pre-cancerous cells had sent me into an emotional tailspin. As odd as it sounds, I was almost angry that the biopsy came back normal. "Normal' what do you mean normal? I had expended so much emotional energy being upset by even the chance of cancer that I felt cheated. I got that upset over nothing? I was so frustrated that I put Peter and me through this emotional roller coaster just for a thickened uterine lining. It sounds crazy to admit it, but in some ways the cancer diagnosis would have been a relief. Yep – I have it, now let's do surgery and get on with it. Without that surgery I just looked at my uterus as a ticking time bomb.

Once I settled down and really thought about it – I realized this was actually really great news, I did NOT have cancer, and I did have an appointment to discuss all my options with the doctor, so in the meantime, I needed to simply let go and see what happens. Now for someone like me who feels a strong need to control things, letting something go of control feels very unnatural. I used a lot of self-talk to calm myself down, and an occasional glass of wine or perhaps a tangerine-watermelon margarita (perhaps the greatest invention known to man).

I was still bleeding, but not as much. I had 4 weeks left of my summer vacation, including a trip I had planned to Texas to see my brother and another trip that would consist of a lazy week of reading and sunbathing in Las Vegas while Peter worked.   I was focusing really hard at appreciating being 'normal', whatever that was.

I also had some plans to kick-start to my weight loss goals. Everything I had read concerning the endometrial issues talked about the need to lose weight and how obesity is one of the risk factors.

So I needed to relax first, then do some serious exercise for my brain AND MY BODY. It sure sounded like a good plan. And hey - this might be the first and only time that I want to celebrate being 'normal'.

I spent the next week relaxing, reading, sunbathing and not thinking at all about my uterus! I had my appointment with the Doctor, so I wrote a full page of questions and concerns to discuss. I was stuck in a very difficult dilemma, the progesterone actually did stop all that bleeding, but I didn't want to stay on it because of all the risk factors. Having a significant family history of breast cancer, I know supplemental hormones are not a good choice for me. Besides, did I mention all of the insanely horrible side-effects listed on the prescription information flier, this stuff can be seriously awful? Bleed constantly or take horrible medicine - either choice did not sound good. Is there a door number three?

I met with the doctor and I must have seemed like a basket case. She was very calm and reassuring, and she did patiently explain the difference between a D&C and an ablation. She then said I would need a referral to a doctor that could do the ablation, because it is not something she does. I would need a gynecologist. The big problem was how long it would take to get into seeing a gynecologist, as most of them were booked for several weeks. I was really hoping to get this taken care of before school started, but it was looking less and less like that would be happening.

I spent several days trying to get an appointment, and could not find a single doctor that could see me in under two weeks. I was so frustrated, I was in tears. I called my doctor's office and asked for help; within one day they had secured me an appointment with a doctor who was close by and willing to see me in just a few days. I was so grateful. The gynecologist office they referred me to was amazing.

It was a bit disconcerting when I entered their office, I was obviously the only woman over 40 in the place, and there were lots of adorable pregnant and newly delivered moms. I came in unsure of what to expect, and a very sweet physician's assistant sat down with me with me to see what was going on. She patiently listened while I explained the saga of my summer, the spotting, the shortened period cycles, the thickened lining, the biopsy, the out of control bleeding and the horrible hormone pills. What happened next was miraculous; she didn't look at me like I was a lunatic, she actually shared that she had a similar experience and that we would get this figured out right away. I know for some of you reading this, your experience was nothing like mine. Women have told me about seeing numerous doctors and not having a single one that will listen to them. I have been so lucky in that regard. In terms of female health – I strongly believe that seeing a female doctor is just better. A male doctor cannot truly empathize with their female patients.

It was tremendously reassuring that this woman understood my fear and had even experienced it herself. The first thing she wanted to do was check and see how thick the lining was and if the hormones had many any difference.   I assumed this meant another week and another doctor's office, but she calmly walked me down the hallway to another office right there in the same building, where another very lovely staff member apologetically performed another pelvic ultrasound and transvaginal ultra sound. Yup folks, another awkward and uncomfortable procedure (by this time I had stopped even counting how many times someone had been putting something into my most private area). But this time at least, I was more prepared for it.

When I was finished I went back into the waiting room, and sat there until the physician's assistant brought me back into the exam room to share the results and make a plan. Well, the good news was, the lining had reduced quite a bit from the hormones. My body was simply producing too much estrogen (darn you Mom for being so fertile) and if I went off the hormones the buildup would likely happen again. She suggested scheduling an ablation, and said there was a good chance that after the procedure I wouldn't have any more periods. That sounded fantastic, especially after the last few months of menstrual hell I had been through. I would need to meet with the surgeon who would do the procedure, but we could get it done before school started. I was so happy about the latter, that it took a little bit for me to register the idea that I was meeting with a surgeon...a surgeon, did this mean it was something actually serious, surgery!

I left their office two hours later with reassurances that my lining was significantly reduced, that it was likely not any form of cancer or hyperplasia and I left with an appointment for meeting the surgeon and a scheduled ablation appointment the week before school started. I was so impressed. I wish I could have done all of this at the beginning of the summer so I would have actually enjoyed the beach and pool for my two months off.

After the initial meeting with the surgeon, I felt comfortable with her and she was very thorough. She explained the procedure, it would be done in their office, I would be under anesthesia and she would basically scrap out all the excess in my lining and then put a metal mesh onto the lining of my uterus, which would then be electrified, in hopes of essentially creating scar tissue that would prevent future build up. Yes folks – I was going to have an electrified uterus. I was pretty angry at my uterus at that point – so sentencing my uterus to electrocution seemed like a fair response to me. She did request that I get the follow-up procedure for the Essure that I had never gotten 4 years ago when I had the Essure implanted. She wanted this prior to the procedure, just to be sure there were no complications and there was no chance I would become pregnant after the ablation – which apparently is a big no-no.

Adding to my extensive resume of gynecological procedures that summer, I made my appointment to have a hysterosalpingogram (HSG), which is typically performed three months after your Essure procedure to confirm whether or not the fallopian tubes are permanently blocked. I have to say that was an exceptionally yucky experience. Once again I am in one of those embarrassing and ill-fitting medical gowns (I really should have invested in one of my own at that point). I climbed up on an ominous looking table in a large X-ray room and put my feet into the now all too familiar stirrups and then a not so pleasant doctor (yes – it was a man, female doctors have a much better empathy for these type of procedures) began to thread a small tube into my uterus. This was not especially comfortable, not only because the male doctor seemed oblivious to my need for any sense of reassurance, let alone privacy, but the tube had to pass through a tiny opening in my cervix to get to my uterus, which was not a very comfortable feeling. At this point they basically fill your uterus with a dye, and yes you are awake, and they x-ray to see if the dye stays in the uterus or if it goes up into the fallopian tubes, which it should not if the Essure has successfully blocked them. Well the good news is that the Essure is working properly, my spring-loaded uterus is performing just right – there will be no babies in my future, unless they are grandchildren. The appointment for the ablation was all set.

Possibly the funniest experience - or the most awful experience of my whole crazy summer happened the night before the ablation procedure - it was our standard back-to-school 'Meet the Teacher night". I had run out of the progesterone pills two day before and decided not to get anymore since the surgery was scheduled for the next day. I had already started bleeding pretty heavily but I thought I was prepared. In addition to the bleeding I began to have more and more hot flashes in the past two weeks, as if my body knew I was planning to get off the hormone pills. Sweat would literally pour off my face during these hot flashes, at least living in Phoenix in the summer, it doesn't seem as out of the norm as it might in other places. Anyhow, I was wearing off-white pants (yes it does seem a tactical error in hindsight) and right in the middle of my second class presentation to eager students and parents I could feel that I was bleeding heavily. I had in a super tampon (changed right before the evening started) and a large pad, but I could tell I was in big trouble. I was trying to stay calm and finish talking with this full room of parents when I began to experience a major hot flash also. Yes, I was standing there bleeding, sweating, and trying so hard to be welcoming to the 50 or so people standing in my classroom. I could see the parents watching me anxiously for any sign that their little prodigy might not be a future President. I tried to make my way towards the door, for a quick exit between classes, but parents kept streaming in. I struggled so hard to concentrate on ancient history – while worrying about making some history of my own….I could just see the red tide slowly spreading between my legs, the screams of horror as the children began to point and faint. It was a moment that I don't think I will ever forget. Somehow I got through the next 10 minutes. I was so thankful when the session was almost over and I spotted another staff member who I asked to stay in my room while I literally ran to the restroom. It was a good thing I did, but of course I had gotten some blood on my pants so I made a futile attempt to pull down my shirt –

which was slightly tight and didn't pull down very far, but somehow I managed to make it work and finished my night. This one experience seems to sum up my entire summer – the chaos and challenges, but I refused to let them interfere with my plans.

I was surprisingly nervous for the actual procedure itself, Peter drove me there and he seemed nervous too, which I am sure added to my tension. The thing I feared the most was the damn IV. I have always had an extreme fear of IV needles. I am sure no one actually likes having an IV put in, but I dread them with an anxiety that borders on pathological. The nurses were a little concerned because my blood pressure was elevated. Was this a surprise to anyone? I was about to have surgery, perhaps I was a little anxious. I tried to reassure them that the fear was more related to getting the stupid IV than the actual procedure, and I guess I convinced them. They checked again and my blood pressure went way down once the dreaded IV was in. After that I don't remember much, I went out like a light and woke up with some mild cramps and a prescription for some Tylenol with codeine for the weekend. Peter once again jumped into action, taking care of my every need and ordering me to go and rest, and given that I was on the aforementioned Tylenol with Codeine, I was more than happy to oblige. I made a point to take it easy for the next few days.

I did not have any real complications from the procedure, I did have some discharge, but after the extensive bleeding I had endured all summer it seemed pretty mild. The first day my uterus felt so heavy and full – like there was a 20lb. brick inside my body, but after a couple of days it was already starting to feel more normal. I felt so lucky to have such a wonderful man like Peter. He had been so caring and attentive, giving me my pills and bringing me drinks. Considering how grumpy and out of sorts I was all through the summer – he endured so much, and he was amazing. I was finally hopeful that after a few weeks my life would return to somewhat normal, without doctor visits, without procedures where people look into or put things into my uterus, and where I didn't have to take those awful hormone pills. They did not agree with my system. AND the extreme bonus that I might not have any more periods at all.

I was dreaming of someday being able to get dressed without pads or panty liners, it may not seem like much of a goal, but I couldn't wait for that day to come. I had been bleeding or spotting since mid-May - yes, that's 4 months straight of bleeding, and even now I had some 'discharge' from the surgery. It wasn't not quite bleeding, but a very lightly pink-tinted watery discharge. According to the doctor I would most likely have this for a few weeks, but possibly up to 6 weeks. Yes, the idea of getting dressed without feeling like I am wearing a diaper sounded miraculous.

After a few more weeks, I wanted to shout from the rooftops, I am NOT bleeding anymore. I was so hopeful that this ablation had done the trick. While I was resting, I did make the mistake of reading Fran Drescher's book "Cancer Schmancer' so now I was even more nervous that maybe there was an issue with the cells in my uterus, I think the doctor took some cells before the ablation and sent them to the lab, but I wasn't 100% sure. I felt fairly confident that if there was anything wrong she would tell me. I did wonder about the chance that the lining would grow back, because we had not dealt with whatever had caused the problem in the first place. It was clear that my extremely thickened lining was not normal and the doctors don't know why it got so thick in the first place.

Now for the bad news, I have decided that this officially sucks, I went through all that turmoil (tests, procedures) to get the ablation, the wondrous cure all for my female problems, but then my stupid period came back. About three months after the procedure, just when I was tricked into hopefully believing that I had said good bye to my monthly visitor forever, it came back. At first I was nervous – "oh no, is this normal" but a quick internet search revealed that periods stop forever in only 50% of the women who have an ablation – a fact that was not made clear to me last summer when discussing options. I think I still would have done the procedure, but I would have had more realistic expectations of the outcome.

Now I not only had the pleasure of having a monthly period, but now I was nervous – my brain was working overtime; is that stupid 'thickened lining' going to come back, am I at risk for cancer, do aliens really exist – okay so I don't actually worry about that last one, I just wanted to see if you were paying attention.

Chapter 9.

Fight like a girl…..if I study harder can I get a good grade?

Oh the joys of getting older. I have always been a surprisingly private person, when I am fearful or stressed out, I rarely go public with my concerns. Even during the worst period of my life, when John (my husband) died and left me to deal with life on my own, as a single parent, I shared my real fears only with my therapist, and on rare occasions with my bff Susan. Keeping it to myself has been a way of life for me. When my mom had her stroke, and when she died, most of my fears stayed inside or sometimes would creep out only in a private journal. With all of that said - I had a new concern and I wanted to shout out about my fear, but my long held 'privacy rule' kept me from reaching out.

Fear, it creeps up and grows. We all know someone who has had cancer, and likely most of us can name more than one person who has died from it. Cancer is the one thing that can take the strongest person in the world, the bravest soldier, the toughest gang member, and make them tremble with fear. In her autobiography "Cancer Schmancer" actress Fran Dresher does a good job of articulating the irrational thought process that cancer creates.

So much has been in the media about breast cancer. Pink themed - fundraising walks and pink ribbons are an iconic piece of our culture today, but other gynecological cancers are rarely talked about. For some reason a breast is okay to discuss, but a uterus is simply not appropriate for polite conversation. Adding to the cancer hysteria already building inside of me, is the shame of my private parts being part of a public conversation. Let's face it, no one wants their uterus to be 'outed' as the source of those killing cells. I'm not sure why boobs are acceptable for being a source of cancer, but a uterus simply is not okay. There is no national group specifically for Uterine/Endometrial cancer.

As women we need to help with awareness of Uterine and other gynaecological cancers. There is more to being a woman than having breasts. Being aware of the risks, getting checked out when something is wrong, being brave enough to face whatever happens – that is fighting like a girl.

According to the American Cancer society, each year, approximately 35,000 women in the United States get uterine cancer. It is the fourth most common cancer in women in the United States and it is the most commonly diagnosed gynecologic cancer. I found this surprising, because we hardly ever hear about uterine cancer, or really any gynecological cancers. If you aren't familiar with gynecological cancers, there are five kinds and they include cervical, ovarian, uterine, vaginal, and vulvar cancers.

When they find evidence of cancer, doctors give the cancer cells a grade, which indicates the severity of the cancer. Remember how I said I was a rule follower, when I was so nervous about having cancer, I wondered how I could get a better grade? Could I do some sort of extra credit? Was there a test I had to study for? If there was, I would promise to cram all night long. Well, being a good student, even though I wasn't diagnosed, I decided to study the stages and grades of uterine cancer.

Treatment for endometrial cancer depends on the size, stage, and grade of the cancer. The stage determines the extent of cancer growth in and beyond the uterus. With a little research on Web MD, I was able to figure out some basic terminology.

Tis (Carcinoma in situ) cancer is found only in one area of the uterus and only in a few layers of cells.

T1 (Stage I) contained in the uterus. It has not spread to the cervix.

T1a (Stage IA) in the lining of the uterus or has spread into less than one-half of the muscle tissue of the uterus.

T1b (Stage IB) spread to one-half or more of the myometrium.

T2 (Stage II) spread from the uterus to the cervix but has not spread outside the uterus.

T3a (Stage IIIA) on the outer surface of the uterus, or in the ovaries or fallopian tubes.

T3b (Stage IIIB) spread into the tissue layers of the vagina.

T4 (Stage IVA) spread into the bladder or rectum.

The grade of endometrial cancer refers to how the cancer cells look under a microscope. Knowing the grade can help your doctor decide which treatment options are best for you. Endometrial cancer cells are described as well-differentiated, moderately differentiated, or poorly differentiated. Differentiation is a term used to describe how clearly the cancer cells can be distinguished from the surrounding normal tissues and how normal or abnormal the cells look.[1]

GX. Grade cannot be assessed

G1: Well-differentiated

G2: Moderately differentiated

G3-G4: Poorly differentiated or undifferentiated

For my story at least so far, I have not had cancer (unless you count a few small skin cancer areas that have been removed), but I know it is still a very real possibility for me. One of my great concerns is that other than unusual bleeding, there are no distinct signs for uterine cancer except for possible pain with urination (which I'm sure is easy to confuse with a simple UTI) and pelvic pain,

---

[1] http://www.webmd.com/cancer/stage-and-grade-of-endometrial-cancer

which seems very generic and difficult to use as an indication of cancer. Other than bleeding or discharge, there is no way to know if something is wrong. There are no simple and reliable ways to test for uterine cancer in women who do not have any signs or symptoms. _Your annual Pap test does not screen for uterine cancer._

According to the Foundation for Women's Cancer the Primary Risk Factors for uterine cancer include; estrogen use without progesterone, diabetes, hypertension, Tamoxifen use, later age of menopause, family history and obesity. I found this list to be utterly unhelpful, it seems like other than trying to control my weight, there is basically nothing I can do to lower my risk factor, and since my uterus has decided not to behave well, I have no way of knowing if uterine cancer is really something I need to worry about. If I were to jump on my soapbox right now, I would urge for more research dollars to study women's health issues and particularly gynecological cancers, but since I would be asking the same men who think a transvaginal ultrasound is a good idea, it might not work out so well.

I was fortunate enough to speak with some women who had gone through uterine cancer. Many of them talked about how this diagnosis caught them completely off-guard. One woman shared "Until I became a member of the club, I never really thought about it being out there. We need to recognize **all** types of Cancer. We need to start representing all types of cancer as well not just recognizing breast cancer awareness."

For most women I spoke to, the shock of being diagnosed was the hardest part, "I hadn't been ready to admit even to myself that I'm a cancer patient. The words are very hard to say out loud". Everyone I talked to wanted to share the same idea, "The biggest message I can give to any one is, if you are in menopause and have any bleeding, tell your doctor, and have it checked out.

I had a history of endometrial hyperplasia for many years but the problem had gone away."

I feel so fortunate to have a great support system like Peter. Other women shared with me how grateful they were for their support as well, "My family stuck by me and showed me that this disease was not the end but just a beginning of the strength I had to become the woman I am today."

Chapter 10.

No Womb at the Inn – a

hysterectomy

There were some days, bleeding and cramping, where I envied my dog because she had been spayed. Now I must say, I love my children beyond measure, and that I know without question that the one thing I did in this life that was truly worthwhile was giving birth to those two amazing young women, but I also know there are literally thousands of women who will would agree with me that a uterus can be a mean and nasty little organ, creating pain and havoc. Despite the difficulties a uterus can bring, the idea of removing your uterus can be troublesome. I have always believed that all of your parts were there for a purpose and that messing around with removing stuff might not be a good idea. After struggling with so many issues caused by my misbehaving uterus, I was willing to make an exception to that rule – just get it out once and for all.

According to the CDC, in the United States, approximately **600,000** hysterectomies are performed each year, and the procedure is the second most frequently performed major surgical procedure among reproductive-aged women. An estimated 20 million U.S. women have had a hysterectomy. For now I am not part of that statistic, but if my bleeding issues return, I will likely get a hysterectomy also. With that in mind I began doing some research on hysterectomies.

There are three main types of hysterectomy: Partial, subtotal, or supracervical - which removes just the upper part of the uterus and the cervix is left in place, Total - which removes the whole uterus and the cervix, and Radical - which removes the whole uterus, the tissue on both sides of the cervix, and the upper part of the vagina. This is usually done when there is cancer present. If you have a total hysterectomy you will enter into menopause immediately, which can be quite a challenge (see Chapter 7 for more details on the exciting menopause symptoms that you will get to enjoy all at once).

There are several different ways that your doctor might perform a hysterectomy, depending on your health history and the reason for your surgery.

- Abdominal hysterectomy is done through a 5- to 7-inch incision, in the lower part of your belly. The cut may go either up and down, or across your belly, just above your pubic hair and it leaves a lovely scar as a souvenir.

- Vaginal hysterectomy is done through a cut in the vagina. The doctor will take your uterus out through this incision and close it with stitches.

- Laparoscopic hysterectomy is done with a laparoscope, an instrument with a thin, lighted tube and small camera that allows your doctor to see your pelvic organs. Your doctor will make three to four small cuts in your belly and insert the laparoscope and other instruments. He or she will cut your uterus into smaller pieces and remove them through the incisions. While this sounds disgusting, the smaller incision leaves a much smaller scar.

- Laparoscopically assisted vaginal hysterectomy is where your doctor removes your uterus through the vagina. The laparoscope is used to guide the procedure.

- Robotic-assisted surgery is where your doctor uses a robot to do the surgery through small cuts in your belly, much like a laparoscopic hysterectomy. Although it sounds very space-age, it is usually done when a patient has cancer or is very overweight and vaginal surgery is not safe.

Most women that I know, myself included, are so busy worrying about everyone else in their life that they rarely take the time to take care of themselves. Recovering from a hysterectomy takes time. Depending on the type of surgery that you had, recovery can take anywhere from 3-4 weeks (for Vaginal or Laparoscopic surgery) to 4 to 6 weeks (for abdominal surgery. You should get plenty of rest and not lift heavy objects for a full 6 weeks after surgery, which is a great excuse to have someone else do the laundry and take out the garbage for a change. Realizing that most of you, like me, are wives and mothers (and really some days are those two roles any different?) it is extremely hard to focus on recovering from surgery and not over-doing it According to the experts, about 6 weeks after either surgery, you should be able to take tub baths and resume sexual intercourse. Research has found that women with a good sex life before hysterectomy can maintain it after the surgery. Of course that same research doesn't indicate what women with lousy sex lives should do.

Chapter 11.

Okay – now what?

For me, the biggest lesson in this whole crazy misadventure has been the need to live in the moment and to accept where I am at in my life. I also learned the importance of listening to my body & trusting my intuition. I know so much more about my uterus than I ever thought I would, but it's important to know about my own body and how it works. That's why I wanted to write this book, to share what I learned with other women. I urge my fellow menopausal sisters, don't keep this information to yourself. Don't suffer in silence. I am grateful that my biopsy was negative for cancer, but I still have to be vigilant, I could still have problems in the future. Breasts may get all the attention, but we need to make sure we don't ignore our uterus, even a mean spirited one like mine.

Here are some great websites that I found while doing my own research, I hope they can help you too:

http://www.womentowomen.com/menopause/uterine hyperplasia.aspx

http://www.cancer.gov/cancertopics/types/endometrial

http://www.ncbi.nlm.nih.gov/pubmedhealth/PMH0001908/

http://www.cancer.org/cancer/endometrialcancer/index

http://www.acog.org/~/media/For%20Patients/faq147.pdf?dmc=1&ts=20120630T1709113045

http://www.womentowomen.com/menopause/uterine hyperplasia.aspx

http://www.dailystrength.org/c/Uterine-Cancer/support-group

http://www.doctoroz.com/blog/lauren-streicher-md/endometrial-ablation-halt-hemorrhage

I also highly recommend the book *Cancer Schmancer* by Fran Drescher

http://www.cancerschmancer.org

Author's Note:

If you enjoyed my book, please take a minute to write a review on Goodreads or Amazon. I would love to hear your comments or suggestions. Your input is extremely valuable to me and to potential readers.

Thanks,
Laurie WJN

www.ingramcontent.com/pod-product-compliance
Lightning Source LLC
Chambersburg PA
CBHW020525290526
45786CB00002B/761